NATURAL ACNE TREATMENT

DR MIRIAM KINAI

ISBN: 1490488677

ISBN-13: 978-1490488677

CONTENTS

ACKNOWLEDGMENTS

I would like to express my sincere gratitude to everyone who contributed in one way or another to the development of this publication.

I would especially like to thank http://www.zazzle.com/ChristianArtGifts for their photographs.

1

DIET THERAPY

Dietary measures that can be used to manage acne include:

1.

Eat Foods With A Glycemic Index Less Than 70

Acne has been called diabetes of the skin due to the relationship between blood sugar levels and acne eruptions.

Therefore, avoid foods with high glycemic indexes like candy, white bread, French fries, mashed potatoes, white flour cakes and doughnuts because they make the blood glucose sugar levels rise rapidly. This rise makes the pancreas produce more insulin in order to regulate the blood glucose level.

The resultant increased insulin level also stimulates the oil glands of the skin to produce sebum (oil) which, if in excess, contributes to clogging the skin pore and the development of whiteheads and blackheads.

Therefore, increase your consumption of low glycemic index foods and preferably those with a glycemic index of less than 70 reduce.

Foods with a glycemic index of less than 20 include:

Peanuts, Broccoli, Cucumber, Green beans, Spinach, Tomatoes

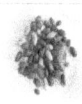 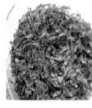 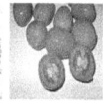

Foods with a glycemic index of 20- 30 include:

Cherries, Soy milk

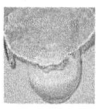

Foods with a glycemic index of 30- 40 include:

Whole wheat spaghetti, Apples, Pears

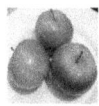

Foods with a glycemic index of 40-50 include:

All bran cereal, Oranges, Pineapple juice, Multi grain bread

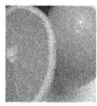

Foods with glycemic index of 50- 60 include:

Bananas, Sweet potato, Oat bran, Brown rice, Popcorn, Mangoes

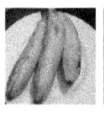 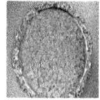 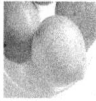

Foods with a glycemic index of 60- 70 include:

Whole meal bread

***

2.

Increase Food Rich in Zinc

Zinc is one of the most important beauty minerals since it is required for collagen formation, wound healing and possibly for helping regulate the activity of the sebaceous (oil) glands.

Zinc also aids the absorption of vitamin A which is another key nutrient for healthy skin.

Food sources of zinc include egg yolks, fish, liver, meat, soybeans, nuts, sunflower seeds and whole grains.

***

3.

Increase Foods Rich in Chromium

Chromium helps pimples heal quickly. It also helps with the metabolism of glucose.

Food sources of chromium include brown rice, meat and whole grains.

***

4.

Increase Foods Rich in Essential Fatty Acids

Essential fatty acids (EFAs) which include the anti-inflammatory omega 3 fatty acids and the omega 6 fatty acids, help in tissue repair as well as in keeping the skin soft and smooth.

Good dietary sources include oily fish like salmon, halibut, mackerel, tuna, anchovies, sardines and shad.

Other good sources of omega 3 fatty acids include avocados, soybeans and soybean oil, sunflower seeds, pumpkin seeds and chia seeds as well as vegetable oils like canola and olive oil.

***

5.

Increase Foods Rich in Antioxidants

Antioxidants like vitamins A, C, E and the mineral selenium protect the skin by neutralizing free radicals from UV radiation, pollution and cigarette smoke which damage the skin. Perfect food sources of antioxidants include:

a) Vitamin A - red bell peppers, mangoes, carrots, cantaloupes, sweet potatoes. These red-to-yellow colored fruits and vegetables contain beta-carotene which is converted in the body into vitamin A which acts synergistically with the other potent antioxidant selenium.

b) Vitamin C - citrus fruits like oranges, guavas, strawberries, melons, avocados, tomatoes. In addition to protecting the skin, vitamins C also helps reduce acne scarring.

c) Vitamin E – almonds, dark green vegetables, avocados, sunflower seeds, eggs and vegetable oils like olive oil, sunflower oil, canola oil and maize oil. In addition to protecting the skin, vitamins E also helps reduce acne scarring.

d) Selenium – meat, garlic, onions, nuts like almonds and brazil nuts.

***

6.

Increase Garlic Intake

Garlic in addition to providing selenium also helps fight infection by enhancing the immune system's functions. You can cut up the raw garlic cloves into small pieces and swallow them with water as you would tablets. Or you can roast them then swallow them. You can also squeeze the juice from the garlic and drink it. Ingest garlic with fresh parsley to minimize its odor.

Due to the potentially clinically significant herb-drug interactions, do not take garlic if you are taking blood thinners such as warfarin, diabetes medications, high blood pressure medications, antiplatelet agents and before surgery.

***

7.

Increase Turmeric Intake

Turmeric is a yellow spice which is used to flavor food. It is also a potent antioxidant with anti- inflammatory properties. Avoid using turmeric if you have ulcers, gall stones and bile duct obstruction.

***

8.

Increase Water Intake

Water helps hydrate the skin from within and keep it healthy. Therefore, drink at least 8 glasses of pure water every day. If you are not used to the taste of water, add ice cubes to drinks like natural fruit juices and dairy-free smoothies to increase your water intake. You can also increase your water intake by eating foods with a high water content like watermelons and cucumbers.

***

9.

Avoid Iodide Rich Foods

Avoid foods that are rich in iodides like iodized table salt, shell fish, seaweed and kelp powder. This is because dietary iodides are excreted from the body through the oil glands and they may contribute to flare up due to impactions.

Substitute the iodized salt with sea salt which has a lower iodine content.

***

10.

Avoid Cow's Milk

Cow's milk has long been suspected to contribute to the development of acne for many years. This is due to its high calcium content, hormonal load and the fact that it contributes to production of excess sebum by the skin's oil glands.

Therefore replace cow's milk, and other dairy products, with soy milk that is fortified with calcium as well as other dietary sources of calcium like spinach.

***

11.

Avoid Sunflower, Safflower and Corn Oil

As you increase your intake of omega 3 fatty acids, keep in mind that eating foods which have more omega 6 fatty acids than omega 3 can cause a form of imbalance that makes the skin cells to stick together and clog the pores. Perfect examples of foods with more omega 6s than 3s include sunflower, safflower and corn oil.

***

12.

Identify and Avoid Trigger Foods

The following foods are suspected to trigger acne:

1. Trans fats which are found in processed foods

2. Caffeine

3. Spicy foods

4. Dairy foods like milk, cheese

5. Processed foods which usually have a high glycemic index and are rich in trans fats

6. Alcohol

7. Soda

8. Cigarette smoke

To identify your trigger foods, keep a food diary so that you can record everything you ate during the 24 hour period that preceded an acne flare up.

* * * * *

2

SUPPLEMENTS

Nutritional supplements that can help treat acne include:

1.

Omega 3 Fatty Acids

These essential fatty acids (EFAs) help in tissue repair as well as in keeping the skin soft and smooth. They also aid in reducing inflammation.

Consider taking a fish oil supplement if you are not eating adequate amounts of cold water fish like sardines and mackerel as well as flaxseed oil, soya oil, canola oil, pumpkin and sunflower seeds.

***

2.

Evening Primrose Oil

Evening primrose oil provides essential fatty acids. 500 mg taken three times a day can help with the management of acne.

***

3.

Zinc

If you are unable to get adequate zinc from your diet, consider taking 30-50 mg Zinc each day to assist with the skin's healing process.

***

4.

Vitamin E

If you are unable to get adequate vitamin E from your diet, consider taking 400 IU Vitamin E daily.

***

5.

Garlic Supplements

Garlic supplements are vital if you cannot tolerate the odor or fresh garlic.

***

5.

Daily Multivitamin

Take one multivitamin, multimineral supplement every day. This supplement should contain:

a) Vitamin A or beta carotene - a powerful antioxidant which is essential for the skin's maintenance and repair.

b) B complex vitamins - include B1, B2, B3, B5, B6 and B12 which are useful for preventing skin disorders and maintaining healthy skin.

c) Vitamin C - essential for collage repair

d) Vitamin E - enhances tissue repair

e) Zinc - aids in healing of tissue

f) Chromium - aids tissue healing

g) Selenium - a vital antioxidant

3

HERBS

Herbs that are used for the natural treatment of acne include:

1.

Neem

Neem is a natural acne remedy that is extracted from crushed neem seeds. It is an effective skin antiseptic which kills bacteria and soothes inflammation without further irritating the skin. Apply it to the blemishes or use soaps, cleansers or moisturizers which contain it.

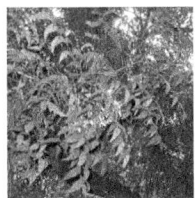

***

2.

Calendula

Calendula is obtained from the plant Calendula officinalis, which is also known as pot marigold. It is a soothing agent which reduces inflammation when applied to the skin.

***

3.

Aloe Vera

Aloe vera has anti-inflammatory properties and acts as a soothing balm for inflamed skin. It also stimulates cell regeneration and is vital for healing. Since it is over 90% water, it is also an excellent oil free moisturizer.

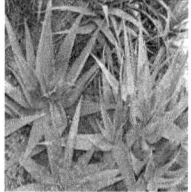

***

4.

Chamomile

Chamomile is soothing to the skin and has anti-inflammatory activity. It also helps in eliminating blackheads by helping open up the pores.

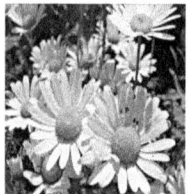

***

5.

Turmeric

Turmeric is a potent antioxidant with anti- inflammatory properties when it is taken by mouth as a food spice.

When applied on the skin, turmeric has antiseptic properties which are useful for clearing acne.

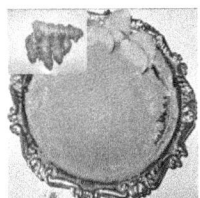

***

6.

Cinnamon

Cinnamon is a spice that has antibacterial, anti-inflammatory and anti-oxidant effects. When the powder is used to form a treatment paste, it also has an exfoliating effect since it helps remove the dead surface skin cells. Cinnamon is therefore very useful for managing acne.

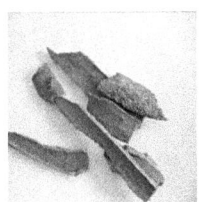

***

7.

Witch Hazel

Witch hazel is an astringent which tightens skin pores and removes excessive oils. It also has healing properties.

***

8.

Garlic

Garlic when taken by mouth helps fight infection by enhancing the immune system's functions.

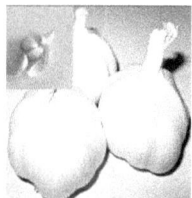

***

OTHER FOOD ITEMS

9.

Pineapple

Pineapple has natural enzymes which remove the dead skin surface cells without causing irritation.

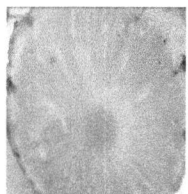

***

10.

Papaya or Pawpaw

Papaya or pawpaw has natural enzymes which exfoliate and remove the dead skin surface cells without irritating the skin.

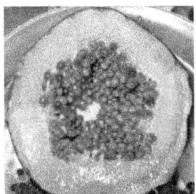

***

11.

Lemon

Lemon contains natural acids which aid in exfoliation and lightening dark acne scars. It can also be used as a toner for oily skin.

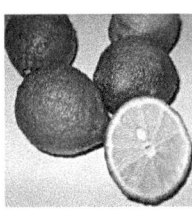

***

12.

Cucumber

Cucumber contains natural astringents which can be used to tone the skin.

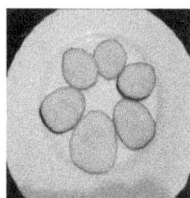

***

13.

Honey

Honey has antiseptic activity which is useful for controlling bacteria. It also softens and moisturizes the skin.

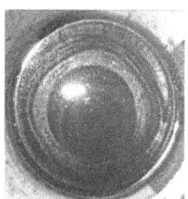

* * * * *

4

ESSENTIAL OILS

Aromatherapy is the use of essential oils for their healing benefits. Each essential oil has a unique scent and effect on the mind and body. Essential oils that are used to treat acne include:

1.

Tea Tree Essential Oil

Tea tree essential oil is extracted from the tea tree leaves. It has powerful antiseptic activity which is useful for killing bacteria and controlling blemishes.

A study conducted at the Royal Prince Alfred proved that a 5% tea tree gel is effective for the treatment of mild to moderate acne.

Tea Tree Essential Oil Safety Information

1. It may be irritating on sensitive skins.

2. It may cause sweating when used in high concentrations. Maximum recommended level is 0.1%.

3. Do not use it alone for more than 2-3 months as it may lead to sensitization.

***

2.

Lavender Essential Oil

Lavender Essential Oil is extracted from lavender flowers. It promotes skin regeneration and has antiseptic and anti-inflammatory properties as well as a calming effect on the mind.

Lavender Essential Oil Safety Information

1. Do not use it in pregnancy especially the first 3 months.

2. Do not use it if you are breastfeeding.

3. Do not use it on young children as it may cause breast development in boys (gynaecomastia) and girls (pre-pubescent breast development).

4. Avoid it if you have low blood pressure as you may feel drowsy after using it.

5. Do not use it alone for more than 2-3 months as it may lead to sensitization.

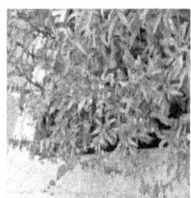

***

3.

Lemon Essential Oil

Lemon essential oil is extracted from the lemon fruit peel and has antiseptic properties.

Lemon Essential Oil Safety Information

1. Do not use it if skin will be exposed to sunlight or UV rays in 12-24 hours as it is phototoxic.

2. Do not use it if you have low blood pressure.

3. It may irritate sensitive skin.

4. Do not use it if you are allergic to lemons.

5. Do not use it alone for more than 2-3 months as it may lead to sensitization.

***

Aromatherapy Acne Treatment Recipes

The first step in using essential oils to treat acne is to do a patch test. To do this, simply add three drops of the essential oil to 5 ml (1 teaspoon) of a carrier oil like jojoba or sweet almond or olive oil and apply the mixture to the inner aspect of your elbow.

Bandage the area and wait for 24 hours to see if you will develop rashes or itchiness or swelling or any other sign of an allergic reaction. If you do, do not use that essential oil.

If you do not develop an allergic reaction, you can use that essential oil to make an acne treatment blend.

A simple "Acne Treatment Blend" can be made by mixing 20 drops of Lavender essential oil, 30 drops of Lemon essential oil and 30 drops of Tea tree essential oil in a dark bottle.

We will refer to this mixture as the "Acne Treatment Blend" in our recipes. If you do not have the three essential oils, you can simply use the one that you have. Therefore if the recipe says, "Add 12 drops of the Acne Treatment Blend", you simply add 12 drops of the essential oil that you have.

Medically Proven Acne Treatment Gel.

A study conducted at the Royal Prince Alfred proved that a 5% tea tree gel is effective for the treatment of mild to moderate acne. This 5% gel can be made by 5 ml of tea tree essential oil to 95 ml of pure aloe vera gel.

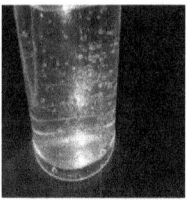

Honey Face Cleanser.

Mix 3 teaspoons of honey with 2 teaspoons of yogurt and add 5 drops of the "Acne Treatment Blend". Massage the mixture onto the blemishes and rinse off with warm water.

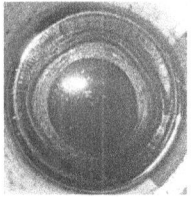

Clay Face Mask.

Add 3 drops of the "Acne Treatment Blend" to 1 teaspoon (5 ml) of fuller's earth clay (bentonite or green clay). Mix with 1 teaspoon of honey and 1 teaspoon of water. Apply it to the face and let it set. Rinse off after 15 minutes with warm water.

Facial Steamer.

Add 50 drops of the "Acne Treatment Blend" (or the number or drops recommended by the manufacturer) to one cup (8 oz or 250 ml) of water and put it on your facial steamer or sauna.

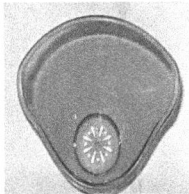

Facial Toner.

Add 20 drops of the "Acne Treatment Blend" to 3 ½ fl ounces or 100 ml of distilled water and use it as you facial toner.

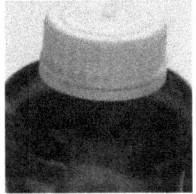

Facial Massage Oil.

Add 20 drops of the "Acne Treatment Blend" to ½ cup (4 oz or 125 ml) of jojoba to create a healing facial massage oil.

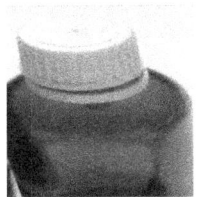

Face Compress.

Add 25 drops (1.25 ml or ¼ teaspoon) of the "Acne Treatment Blend" to ½ cup (4 oz or 125 ml) of warm water, dip your hand towel or bath cloth or sponge in it and wipe your face body with it after stepping out of the shower or bath tub.

Mini Acne Treatment Oil.

Add 2 drops of the "Acne Treatment Blend" essential oil to 10 ml of jojoba and put it in a small bottle that can fit into your purse to pocket. Carry it with you to dab at any fresh breakouts with a cotton bud at least thrice a day.

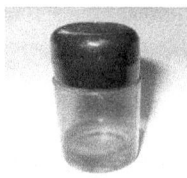

Aromatherapy Bath.

Create a healing bath by dispersing 12 drops of the "Acne Treatment Blend" in your warm bath water. This is especially beneficial if you have back acne.

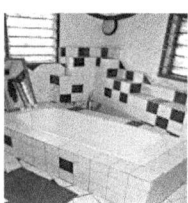

Bath Gel.

Add 50 drops (2.5 ml or ½ teaspoons) of the "Acne Treatment Blend" to one cup (8 oz or 250 ml) of unscented bath gel or liquid soap to create a healing bath gel.

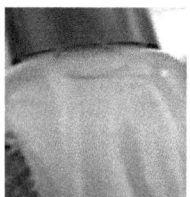

Bath Tea.

Mix 2 cups of herbs like lavender flowers and neem leaves with 15 drops of the "Acne Treatment Blend" and 1 cup of sea salt. Put the mixture in an air tight jar or you can add a scoopful of the mixture into a cotton bath tea bag and store the filled bath tea bags in the air tight jar.

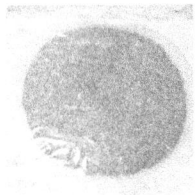

Body Wrap.

Add 20 drops of the "Acne Treatment Blend" to 3 oz or 100 ml of distilled water and spray it on your towel. Wrap your body in the towel and then wrap a plastic sheet around yourself and relax for 20 min before you unwrap yourself.

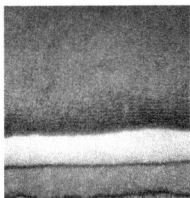

Body Oil.

Add 50 drops (2.5 ml or ½ teaspoons) of the "Acne Treatment Blend" to one cup (8 oz or 250 ml) of jojoba and use it as an after shower body oil. Massage it into your skin after patting it dry but while it is still moist to lock in the moisture and healing benefits of the essential oils. This body oil can also be used as an aromatherapy body massage oil. Do not massage your skin if you have inflammed acne lesions.

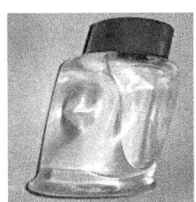

Body Splash.

Add 50 drops (2.5 ml or ½ teaspoons) of the "Acne Treatment Blend" to one cup (8 oz or 250 ml) of distilled water in a spray bottle and use it to spray your face and body whenever you need to refresh.

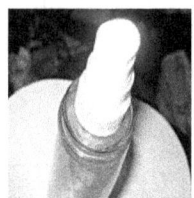

* * * * *

5

LIFESTYLE MODIFICATIONS

Lifestyle modifications that are useful for managing acne include:

1.

Manage Stress

Effective stress management is important for managing acne effectively since a study proved that there is a correlation between high levels of emotional stress levels and more severe acne.

This link between acne and stress is thought to be due to the stress hormone cortisol which results in an increase in the amount of oil that the skin produces. The excess oil produced during stressful periods then contributes to the clogging of the skin pores and the eruption of acne lesions.

If you have acne, it is important to determine if it is stress related so that you can practice relaxation techniques religiously when you are going through stressful periods to prevent breakouts.

To determine if your acne is stress related, examine your face closely during "stressful periods" to see if your acne pimples have increased in number, redness and size and if they last longer. If they do, then your acne is stress related.

If it is stress related acne, practice effective relaxation techniques and deal with the root cause of your stress because if the stress is not managed, it will result in a vicious cycle in which new pimples cause more stress which in turn results in more pimples.

***

2.

Change your Hairstyle

If you have a fringe, change your hairstyle. Keep your hair off your face to prevent it from depositing pore plugging oils on your face.

You should also avoid using oily hair sprays and greasy hair oils that run down to your forehead and clog the pores. Ensure that you also shampoo your hair frequently.

***

3.

Wash your Pillow Case

Your pillow case absorbs the oils and dirt from your hair and face and reapplies them to your face every night as you sleep. This can contribute to plugging pores so keep your sheets and pillow cases pristine.

***

4.

Change your Thinking Pose

If you break out on one cheek, it could be due to the extra pressure from leaning on your chin or cheek with your hand as you think. So, change your thinking pose and keep your hands off your face.

***

5.

Sanitize your Mobile

Clean your mobile phone to remove the bacteria that may promote acne in your cheek area and jaw line.

***

6.

Clean your Equipment

If you must use makeup, wash your brushes and replace the sponges regularly to avoid spreading bacteria. If possible, apply your makeup with clean cotton wool balls that you can dispose off after a single use.

***

7.

Exercise Regularly

Regular exercise is important for treating acne because:

1. It is an effective relaxation technique which reduces stress related acne breakouts.

2. It increases circulation in the skin and results in a healthy glow.

***

8.

Stop Smoking

Quit smoking since it releases toxins and constricts blood vessel thereby restricting the supply of nutrients that are vital for healthy skin. The free radicals in cigarette smoke also damage the skin, resulting in loss of elasticity and wrinkles.

To help you stop smoking, follow the following mnemonic:

S Set a date to stop

T Think about why you want to stop smoking and write down all your reasons.

O Omit places that remind you of smoking from your schedule and avoid people who encourage you to smoke.

P Place obstacles between you and cigarettes by getting rid of all the cigarettes in your house, car and office.

9.

Get Adequate Sleep

Get 7-10 hours of beauty sleep every night to rejuvenate your skin and heal it with your night time acne treatment products.

***

10.

Improve your Spiritual Health

Studies have shown that people of faith recover faster from illnesses and surgery. Therefore begin practicing your faith by giving yourself the following Spiritual Facial each day to ensure a blemish free inner life:

1. Cleanse your spirit by confessing your sins.

2. Tone it by thanking God for your blessings.

3. Steam it with forgiveness to open up your pores and let go of bitterness and vengeance.

4. Apply the mask of salvation to remove all sins from your deepest pores.

5. Spot treat the blemishes of worry and doubt with faith and trusting God.

6. Moisturize it with prayer to keep it radiant, supple and healthy.

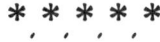

* * * * *

6

EXERCISE PLAN

A balanced exercise plan should combine stretching, weight bearing and aerobic exercises.

If you have been leading a sedentary lifestyle, consult your doctor and nutritionist before making changes to your exercise regimen.

In addition, invest in a good pair of sports shoes that will cushion your feet and redistribute your weight evenly as you walk, jog, jump or run.

If as you exercise, you experience any of the following symptoms, stop exercising at once and consult your doctor: chest pain, pressure or tightness, unusual shortness of breath, pain in the jaw, arm, neck or shoulder, palpitations or skipped heart beats, feeling dizzy or fainting, muscle pain that is more severe than just discomfort.

1.

Stretching Exercises

Stretch for at least 10 minutes each morning and evening and in the warm up and cool down periods just before or right after your exercise sessions.

To stretch correctly you should:

1. Not hold your breath as you stretch. Breathe in and out rhythmically.

2. Never bounce into or out of your stretches. Gently move into and out of the various positions.

3. Hold the stretch position for 10 seconds and gradually increase the duration.

4. Be systematic and begin with the legs as you work your way up the body to the neck or vice versa.

5. Stop stretching if you feel any pain but continue if you experience mild discomfort.

The following is a list of exercises that you can do at home to stretch your entire body.

1. Neck Stretch - Stand with your feet shoulder width apart and your chin on your chest. Rotate your head once clockwise. Return chest to chin and rotate it counter clockwise. Do several rotations. Turn your face to the right, look as far back over your shoulder as you can. Hold for a count of 10. Repeat on opposite side.

2. Chest, Shoulder and Arm Stretch - Stand with your feet shoulder width apart and your knees slightly bent. Clasp your hands behind your back and push them back as far as you can reach. Push your chest forward as far as it can reach. Hold and return to starting position.

3. Side Stretch - Stand straight with your arms raised over your head. Tilt your body to the left side as you stretch your side muscles. Hold. Repeat on the opposite side.

4. Abs, Glutes and Quads Stretch - Stand with your feet together. Reach forward with your right arm. Lift your left leg behind you and grasp your left ankle with your left hand. Lift your left thigh as high as you can or until it is parallel to the ground. Repeat on opposite side.

5. Back Stretch - Lie on your back and pull both knees to your chest. Release them and lower your knees to the right side and then to the left side. Return knees back to chest.

6. Hamstring Stretch - Lie on your back with your legs bent and both feet flat on the floor. Straighten and raise your right leg. Gently pull your right thigh towards your body and hold for a count of 10. Repeat on the opposite side.

2.

Weight Bearing Exercises

To weight train or strength train correctly you should:

a) Not hold your breath or strain as you train.

b) Not exercise the same muscle groups for two consecutive days.

c) Aim for 3 sets of 10 repetitions each.

The following are exercises that you can do at home to strength train your entire body.

1. Overhead Press - (Works shoulders) Sit on a chair; hold a weight (or a full water bottle) in each hand at shoulder level with palms facing forward. Raise your arms straight up over your head. Lower them to shoulder level.

2. Biceps Curl - (Works biceps) Sit on a chair; hold a weight (or a full water bottle) in each hand palms facing forward. Bend your elbow and lift the weight towards your shoulder. Return to starting position and repeat with the other arm.

3. Triceps Dips - (Works triceps) Sit on the edge of a sturdy chair with your back and shoulders straight. Hold the edge of a chair and bend your elbows to form a right angle as you lower your butt off the seat to the floor. Straighten your arms and press back up to raise your butt back to the seat.

4. Push Ups - (Works deltoids, triceps, pectorals) Lie on floor, palms face down, elbows bent next to shoulders. Push up from floor by straightening elbows and contracting abs so that your body forms a straight line from your head to heel (beginners can rest both knees on floor) Lower yourself to floor by bending elbows. Push back up.

5. Simple Straight Crunches - (Works abs) Lie flat on your back; bend knees while keeping your feet flat on the floor. Place your hands on your thighs. Exhale and lift shoulder blades from the floor as you slide your hands up to your knees. Hold for a count of 10. Return to starting position and repeat.

6. Simple Side Crunches - (Works abs) Lie flat on your back; bend knees while keeping your feet flat on the floor. Place your hands on your right thigh. Exhale and lift shoulder blades from the floor as you slide your hands up to your right knee. Hold for a count of 10. Return to starting position and repeat. Do on opposite side.

7. Advanced Straight Crunches - (Works abs) Lie flat on your back; bend your knees until thighs are perpendicular to floor. Place arms crossed over your chest. Exhale, tighten abs and lift shoulder blades from the floor as you reach towards knees. Hold for a count of 10. Return to starting position and repeat.

8. Advanced Side Crunches - (Works abs) Lie flat on your back; bend your knees until thighs are perpendicular to floor. Place arms crossed over your chest. Exhale, tighten abs and lift shoulder blades from floor as you reach towards right knee. Hold for a count of 10. Return to starting position and repeat. Do on opposite side.

9. Leg Lifts - Lie on your back; legs straight; hands under butt. Lift legs 30 cm from the floor. Hold for a count of 10.

10. Lunge - (Works glutes, hamstrings, quadriceps) Stand with feet shoulder width apart, arms at sides. Take a large step forward with your left leg and ensure your left knee is above your left foot. Lower your body to the floor by bending the right knee until right thigh is parallel to the floor and right knee is close to the ground. Squeeze your glutes as you press back up to your starting position. Repeat on opposite side.

11. Squat - (Works your butt and thighs) Stand with your feet parallel and shoulder width apart. Stretch out your hands in front of you. Keeping your abs and butt tight, bend your knees and slowly lower yourself as though you are sitting. Ensure your knees don't extend past your toes. Hold for a count of 10. As your rise, squeeze your glutes.

12. Calf Raises - (Work your calf muscles) Stand with feet together and arms raised above your head. Lift your heels so that you are standing on the balls of your feet/toes. Stand on your toes for a count of 10.

3.

Aerobic Exercises

Aerobic exercises include walking, skipping a rope, jogging (on a treadmill or in the park), cycling or spinning in the gym, swimming, aerobic classes in a gym, sports like tennis and basketball as well as everyday activities like climbing stairs, housework and gardening.

Swimming is a good option especially if you are overweight or obese because it does not put excessive pressure on the joints of the lower limbs.

To reap the most benefits from your aerobic exercise sessions, you should:

1. Exercise for at least 30 min each session

2. Reach your Target Heart Rate (THR) which is calculated by

220 - your age = maximum heart rate (MHR)

MHR x 0.65 = minimum target heart rate (MinTHR)

MHR x 0.80 = maximum target heart rate (MaxTHR)

For example, if you are 40 years old, 220 - 40 years = 180 your maximum heart rate (MHR)

180 (MHR) x 0.65 = 117 your minimum target heart rate (MinTHR)

180 (MHR) x 0.80 = 144 your maximum target heart rate (MaxTHR)

Therefore, as you exercise, you should ensure that your heart rate is between 117 and 144.

To know your heart rate per minute, take your pulse on your wrist or neck for one minute.

The following is a rough guide of target heart rates for different age groups:

If you are 20 years old, your Target Heart Rate (THR) per minute should be 130 - 160

If you are 30 years old, your Target Heart Rate (THR) per minute should be 123 – 152

If you are 40 years old, your Target Heart Rate (THR) per minute should be 117 – 144

If you are 50 years old, your Target Heart Rate (THR) per minute should be 110 – 136

If you are 60 years old, your Target Heart Rate (THR) per minute should be 104 – 128

If you are 70 years old, your Target Heart Rate (THR) per minute should be 97 – 120

If you are 80 years old, your Target Heart Rate (THR) per minute should be 91 – 112

***

Exercise Plan

You can modify this plan to suit your lifestyle and level of activity.

Exercise Activity for Week 1

Day 1

Whole body stretch to warm up

30 min walk at minimum THR

Whole body stretch to cool down

Day 2

Whole body stretch to warm up

10 push ups, 10 triceps dips, 10 crunches

Whole body stretch to cool down

Day 3

Whole body stretch to warm up

30 min walk at minimum THR

Whole body stretch to cool down

Day 4

Whole body stretch to warm up

10 squats, 10 lunges, 10 calf raises, 10 crunches

Whole body stretch to cool down

Day 5

Whole body stretch to warm up

30 min walk at minimum THR

Whole body stretch to cool down

Exercise Activity for week 2

Day 1

Whole body stretch to warm up

30 min walk/ jog at medium THR

Whole body stretch to cool down

Day 2

Whole body stretch to warm up

15 push ups, 15 bicep curls, 15 triceps dips, 15 crunches

Whole body stretch to cool down

Day 3

Whole body stretch to warm up

30 min walk/ jog at medium THR

Whole body stretch to cool down

Day 4

Whole body stretch to warm up

15 squats, 15 lunges, 15 calf raises, 15 crunches

Whole body stretch to cool down

Day 5

Whole body stretch to warm up

30 min walk/ jog at medium THR

Whole body stretch to cool down

Exercise Activity for week 3

Day 1

Whole body stretch to warm up

30 min walk/run maximum THR

Whole body stretch to cool down

Day 2

Whole body stretch to warm up

20 push ups, 20 bicep curls, 20 triceps dips, 20 crunches

Whole body stretch to cool down

Day 3

Whole body stretch to warm up

30 min walk/run maximum THR

Whole body stretch to cool down

Day 4

Whole body stretch to warm up

20 squats, 20 lunges, 20 calf raises, 20 crunches

Whole body stretch to cool down

Day 5

Whole body stretch to warm up

30 min walk/run maximum THR

Whole body stretch to cool down

Exercise Activity for week 4

Day 1

Whole body stretch to warm up

30 min walk/run maximum THR

Whole body stretch to cool down

Day 2

Whole body stretch to warm up

30 push ups, 30 bicep curls, 30 triceps dips, 30 crunches

Whole body stretch to cool down

Day 3

Whole body stretch to warm up

30 min walk/run maximum THR

Whole body stretch to cool down

Day 4

Whole body stretch to warm up

30 push ups, 30 bicep curls, 30 triceps dips, 30 crunches

Whole body stretch to cool down

Day 5

Whole body stretch to warm up

30 min walk/run maximum THR

Whole body stretch to cool down

* * * * *

7

STRESS MANAGEMENT PLAN

Learning and practicing relaxation techniques is a very effective way of managing stress. These relaxation techniques include:

1.

Meditation

Meditation is another effective relaxation technique for coping with stress. To meditate, simply lie down in a quiet place and take several deep breaths. Once your body begins to feel calmer, focus on your inhalation and on the pure oxygen entering your body. As you exhale, envision you whole body relaxing. You can also meditate on Scriptures like **With God all things are possible** (Matthew 19:26) and envisioning your stressful situation resolving miraculously.

***

2.

Abdominal Breathing

Abdominal breathing or deep breathing is one fastest ways of counteracting the body's stress response. It is done by inhaling through your nose until your abdomen rises, holding your breath for a few moments and then exhaling completely through your mouth until your abdomen collapses. This cycle of filling the lungs with air, pausing and then emptying them can be repeated for 15 minutes every day.

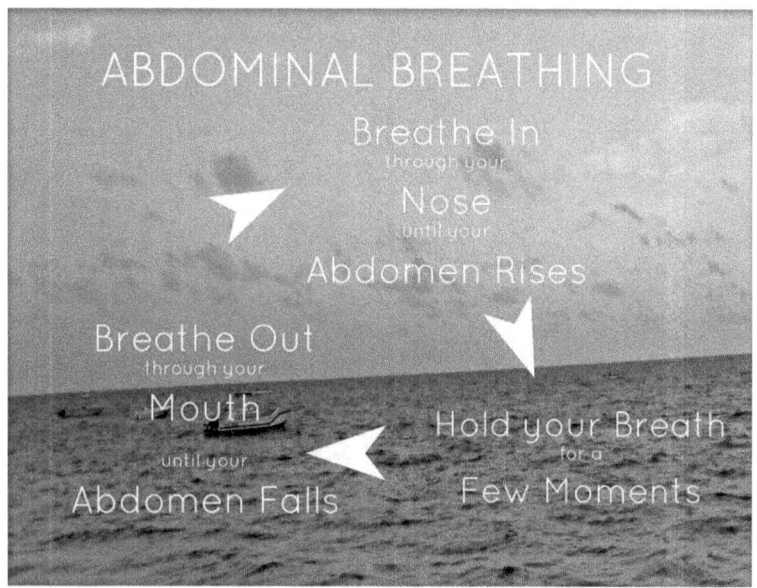

***

3.

Guided Imagery

Guided imagery is another effective relaxation technique. It involves visualizing yourself in a relaxing environment. Therefore close your eyes, take several deep breaths and use your mind's eye to see yourself relaxing on a beach or floating on a cloud or walking through a garden or whichever environment makes you feel relaxed. Use all your senses to immerse yourself in the restful environment by seeing soothing images, smelling appealing scents, hearing calming sounds, tasting and feeling your way through it. After you have enjoyed our visit, bring yourself gently back to reality.

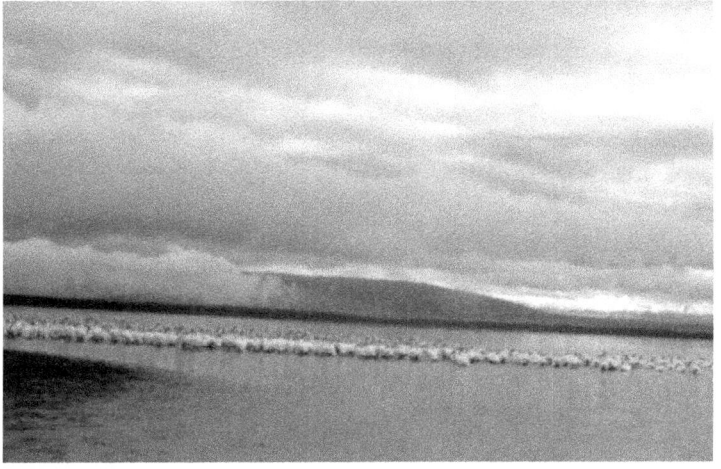

***

4.

Problem Solving Visualization

Visualization can also be used to manage stressful situations. To do this see yourself with your mind's eye in your most stressful situation and then envisioning yourself using various strategies to cope. For example you can imagine yourself dealing with a stressful boss by breathing deeply until you no longer feel distressed by their words or actions.

***

5.

Physical Exercise

When a person is stressed, they tense their muscles. Stretching exercises reduce this muscle tension and help a person feel relaxed.

Aerobic exercises help the body burn circulating stress hormones that contribute to the development of stress related illnesses.

Weight bearing exercises also aid in stress management since they demand concentration and help a person forget their problems.

Therefore engage in regular physical exercises to manage stress.

Relaxing Activities

Other relaxing activities that you can engage in to manage stress include:

1. Journaling since writing down uncensored feelings is a very effective method of catharsis. It is doubly effective when combined with writing lists of things you are thankful for.

2. Listening to calming music.

3. Engaging in hobbies that complement their main job

4. Helping less fortunate members of your society like visiting the sick in hospitals since this takes your mind off your problems

5. Drinking soothing herbal teas like chamomile and passionflower.

6. Eating foods which raise serotonin levels like turkey, salmon, chicken, cheese, chocolate, wholegrain bread.

7. Watching comedy since laughter relieves tension.

8. Spending time with your social support system.

***

Stress Management Plan

Stress Management Plan Week 1

Day 1

1. Abdominal breathing

2. Meditation

3. Physical Exercise

4. Watching Comedy

Day 2

1. Abdominal breathing

2. Meditation

3. Drinking herbal teas and eating serotonin rich foods

4. Watching Comedy

Day 3

1. Abdominal breathing

2. Meditation

3. Physical Exercise

4. Watching Comedy

Day 4

1. Abdominal breathing

2. Meditation

3. Drinking herbal teas and eating serotonin rich foods

4. Watching Comedy

Day 5

1. Abdominal breathing

2. Meditation

3. Physical Exercise

4. Watching Comedy

Day 6 and 7

1. Abdominal breathing 2. Meditation 3. Spending time with your social support system

Stress Management Plan Week 2

Day 1

1. Abdominal breathing

2. Guided imagery

3. Physical Exercise

4. Listening to Music

Day 2

1. Abdominal breathing

2. Guided imagery

3. Drinking herbal teas and eating serotonin rich foods

4. Listening to Music

Day 3

1. Abdominal breathing

2. Guided imagery

3. Physical Exercise

4. Listening to Music

Day 4

1. Abdominal breathing

2. Guided imagery

3. Drinking herbal teas and eating serotonin rich foods

4. Listening to Music

Day 5

1. Abdominal breathing

2. Guided imagery

3. Physical Exercise

4. Listening to Music

Day 6 and 7

1. Abdominal breathing 2. Guided imagery 3. Engaging in Complementary Hobbies

Stress Management Plan Week 3

Day 1

1. Abdominal breathing

2. Problem solving visualization

3. Physical Exercise

4. Journaling and writing gratitude lists

Day 2

1. Abdominal breathing

2. Problem solving visualization

3. Drinking herbal teas and eating serotonin rich foods

4. Journaling and writing gratitude lists

Day 3

1. Abdominal breathing

2. Problem Solving Visualization

3. Physical Exercise

4. Journaling and writing gratitude lists

Day 4

1. Abdominal breathing

2. Problem Solving Visualization

3. Drinking herbal teas and eating serotonin rich foods

4. Journaling and writing gratitude lists

Day 5

1. Abdominal breathing

2. Problem Solving Visualization

3. Physical Exercise

4. Journaling and writing gratitude lists

Day 6 and 7

1. Abdominal breathing 2. Problem Solving Visualization 3. Helping the less fortunate

Stress Management Plan Week 4

Day 1

1. Abdominal breathing

2. Meditation or Guided Imagery or Problem Solving Visualization (choose the one that has been most relaxing for you and practice it regularly)

3. Physical exercise

4. Watching Comedy or Listening to Music or Journaling and writing gratitude lists (choose the one that has been most relaxing for you and practice it regularly)

Day 2

1. Abdominal breathing

2. Meditation or Guided Imagery or Problem Solving Visualization (choose the one that has been most relaxing for you and practice it regularly)

3. Drinking herbal teas and eating serotonin rich foods

4. Watching Comedy or Listening to Music or Journaling and writing gratitude lists (choose the one that has been most relaxing for you and practice it regularly)

Day 3

1. Abdominal breathing

2. Meditation or Guided Imagery or Problem Solving Visualization (choose the one that has been most relaxing for you and practice it regularly)

3. Physical exercise

4. Watching Comedy or Listening to Music or Journaling and writing gratitude lists (choose the one that has been most relaxing for you and practice it regularly)

Day 4

1. Abdominal breathing

2. Meditation or Guided Imagery or Problem Solving Visualization (choose the one that has been most relaxing for you and practice it regularly)

3. Drinking herbal teas and eating serotonin rich foods

4. Watching Comedy or Listening to Music or Journaling and writing gratitude lists (choose the one that has been most relaxing for you and practice it regularly)

Day 5

1. Abdominal breathing

2. Meditation or Guided Imagery or Problem Solving Visualization (choose the one that has been most relaxing for you and practice it regularly)

3. Physical exercise

4. Watching Comedy or Listening to Music or Journaling and writing gratitude lists (choose the one that has been most relaxing for you and practice it regularly)

Day 6 and 7

1. Abdominal breathing

2. Meditation or Guided Imagery or Problem Solving Visualization (choose the one that has been most relaxing for you and practice it regularly)

3. Spending time with your social support system or Engaging in complementary hobbies or Helping the less fortunate (choose the one that has been most relaxing for you and practice it regularly)

###

ABOUT THE AUTHOR

Dr. Miriam Kinai is a medical doctor and freelance health writer/blogger.

You can visit her blog at http://www.MyBlogBookClub.com or follow her on twitter at http://twitter.com/AlmasiHealth

Email enquiries to almasihealthcare@yahoo.com with BOOKS as your subject.

HERBS AND SPICES FOR THE COOK, HEALER AND BEAUTICIAN

Herbs and Spices for the Cook, Healer and Beautician uses color pictures and clear explanations to teach you about more than 70 healing herbs and spices.

You will learn about their:

* Therapeutic (healing) uses

* Drug interactions

* Contraindications (when not to use them)

* Cooking tips

* Beauty tips

*****

INTERNATIONAL GOURMET HERB AND SPICE BLENDS

International Gourmet Herb and Spice Blends teaches you how to prepare exotic herb and spice blends from around the world. You will discover the recipes for:

* Barbecue Rub, Cajun, Apple Pie and Pumpkin Pie Spice Mixes from America

* Pudding Spice Mix from Britain

* 5 Spice Mix from China

* Berbere Spice Mix from Ethiopia

* Curry Powder and Garam Masala from India

* Bouquet Garni, Herbs de Provence and Quatre Epices from France

* Herb Mix from Italy

* Jerk Seasoning from Jamaica

* Shichimi Togarashi from Japan

* Pilau Spice Blend from Kenya

* Chili Powder from Mexico

* Baharat Spice Blend from the Middle East

* Ras El Hanout from Morocco

*****

THE QUICK GOURMET CHEF

The Quick Gourmet is an essential culinary skills cookbook which teaches how to make simple, divine dishes.

You will learn how to make:

* Hot Chocolate Mixes and Drinks

* Hot Chai Tea Mixes and Drinks

* Hot Coffee Mixes and Drinks

* Sensational Smoothies

* Non-Dairy Smoothies

* Chocolate Covered Strawberries

* Chocolate Truffles

* Healthy Chicken Salads

* Healthy Tuna Salads

* Savory Salsas

* Herb Butter

* Cheese Dips and Sauces

* Gourmet Sandwiches

* Perfect Hard Boiled Eggs

* A Cheese Board

* Natural Food Color

*****

HOW TO STYLE AND PHOTOGRAPH FOOD

Regardless of whether you are an aspiring food blogger or you want to make money online selling stock photos, How To Style and Photograph Food, uses color pictures and clear explanations to teach you the food photography tips that can help you improve your digital camera photography skills so that you can begin photographing food like a pro.

You will learn:

* The equipment that you need

* How to set up the lighting

* How to prepare the stage

* How to style the food

* How to shoot the food

*****

HOW TO MAKE NATURAL SKIN CARE PRODUCTS VOLUME 1

How To Make Natural Skin Care Products Volume 1 by Dr Miriam Kinai is filled with recipes for making organic bath and body products for normal, sensitive, oily and dry skin types as well as therapeutic products to manage mature skin, prematurely aging skin, cellulite, eczema, psoriasis, ringworms, dandruff, thinning hair, menopausal symptoms, pre-menstrual tension (PMS), painful periods, arthritis, stress, sadness or depression, mental exhaustion and insomnia.

This book also teaches you the best vegetable oils, essential oils, natural butters and herbs to use when making products for different skin types physical conditions. You will learn how to make:

* Bath bombs

* Bath melts

* Bath salts

* Bath teas

* Body butters

* Body lotions

* Body scrubs

* Healing balms and body creams

* Herb infused oils

* Natural soap

How to Make Natural Skin Care Products Volume 1 will leave you with a clear understanding of how to make bath and beauty products to use in your home or to give as gifts or to sell and make money.

*****

ORGANIC SKIN CARE PRODUCT INGREDIENTS

Organic Skin Care Product Ingredients teaches you about the different natural substances that can be used to create natural bath and beauty products to use in your home or to give as gifts to your loved ones or to sell and make money.

You will learn about:

* Natural butters

* Natural clays

* Natural colorants

* Natural exfoliants

* Natural fragrances

* Natural oils

* Natural preservatives

*****

THE ESSENTIALS OF AROMATHERAPY ESSENTIAL OILS

The Essentials of Aromatherapy Essential Oils by Dr Miriam Kinai teaches you how to use aromatherapy oils to improve your physical, mental and emotional well being.

The author's experience as a medical doctor and clinical aromatherapy practitioner have enabled her to write a highly informative guide for those who want to utilize the healing benefits of these natural plant essences.

You will discover:

* The safety information and therapeutic uses of 18 essential oils

* How to blend essential oils

* The characteristics and uses of 14 carrier oils

* How to Dilute Essential Oils with Carrier Oils

* How to Use Essential Oils

* Cautionary Measures when using Essential Oils

* Numerous Essential Oil Recipes for bath products as well as skin care and hair care products

The Essentials of Aromatherapy Essential Oils will leave you with a clear understanding of how you can safely use aromatherapy essential oils to heal yourself naturally.

*****

CARRIER OILS GUIDE

Carrier Oils Guide teaches you the characteristics, health benefits and uses of commonly used carrier oils. You will learn about:

* Apricot Kernel Oil

* Avocado Oil

* Borage Seed Oil

* Calendula Oil

* Carrot Seed Oil

* Castor Oil

* Evening Primrose Oil

* Fractionated Coconut Oil

* Jojoba

* Olive Oil

* Rosehip Oil

* Sunflower Oil

* Sweet Almond Oil

* Virgin Coconut Oil

* Useful formulas for Diluting Essential Oils with Carrier Oils

*****

MEDICAL AROMATHERAPY FOR HEALTH PROFESSIONALS

Medical Aromatherapy for Healthcare Professionals by Dr Miriam Kinai teaches you how to use essential oils to treat physical diseases and emotional disorders.

The author's experience as a medical doctor and clinical aromatherapy practitioner have enabled her to write a highly informative guide for those who want to utilize the healing benefits of these natural plant essences.

You will discover how to use essential oils to:

* Treat skin diseases like acne, eczema and psoriasis

* Treat other physical diseases like high blood pressure, arthritis, coughs and colds

* Manage mental and emotional conditions like anxiety, depression, anger and stress

* Relieve the symptoms of menopause and premenstrual tension

* Lessen insomnia and impotence

Medical Aromatherapy for Healthcare Professionals is therefore an essential resource for holistic healthcare practitioners like massage therapists, naturopaths and herbalists.

It is also a useful resource for conventional medicine healthcare providers like physicians and nurses who want to begin practicing integrative medicine and for patients who want to improve their health naturally by using aromatherapy oils.

*****

AROMATHERAPY COURSE

Aromatherapy Course by Dr Miriam Kinai tutors you on how to use essential oils to improve your physical, mental and emotional well being.

The author's experience as a medical doctor and clinical aromatherapy practitioner have enabled her to create a highly informative course on how to use these natural plant essences.

You will learn:

* The safety information and therapeutic uses of essential oils like clary sage, eucalyptus, geranium, grapefruit, lavender, lemon, lemongrass, marjoram, orange (sweet), patchouli, peppermint, Roman chamomile, rose, rosemary, sandalwood, spearmint, tea tree and ylang ylang.

* The safety information and therapeutic uses of carrier oils like apricot kernel oil, avocado oil, borage seed oil, calendula oil, carrot seed oil, castor oil, evening primrose oil, fractionated coconut oil, jojoba, olive oil, rosehip oil, sunflower oil, sweet almond oil and virgin coconut oil.

* How to blend essential oils

* How to dilute essential oils with carrier oils

* How to administer essential oils

* How to make natural healing products from numerous aromatherapy recipes

* How to utilize the healing benefits of essentials oils even if you do not have prior training in aromatherapy

The Aromatherapy Course will leave you with a clear understanding of how you can heal yourself and your family naturally by using essentials oils on your body and in your home.

*****

DEALING WITH DEPRESSION NATURALLY

Dealing with Depression Naturally presents a holistic approach to managing depression with natural antidepressants. You will learn how to treat depression with:

* Aromatherapy

* Art therapy

* Christian Biblical principles

* Chromotherapy

* Diet therapy

* Eco-therapy

* Herbal therapy

* Home decor therapy

* Music therapy

* Phototherapy

* Exercise therapy

* Self-Psychotherapy

* Social therapy

* Talk therapy

* Vitamin therapy

* Writing therapy

*****

CHRISTIAN LIFE COACHING HANDBOOK

Christian Life Coaching Handbook offers a Biblical approach to managing different aspects of life.

You will learn:

* Christian anger management

* Christian conflict resolution

* Christian depression treatment

* Christian goal setting

* Christian marital stress management

* Christian stress management

* How to assert yourself

* How to defeat fear

* How to love yourself

* How to overcome shyness

* How to resist temptation

* How to stop being a people pleaser

*****

CHRISTIAN PERSONAL FINANCE

Christian Personal Finance teaches Biblical principles of money management.

You will learn:

* Christian financial stress management from people who were dealing with money stress like the Acts 3 beggar or credit issues like the widow in second Kings.

* Biblical prosperity principles from wealthy men and women of God like Isaac and the Proverbs 31 woman.

* Bible verses to use as spiritual warfare prayers and as Christian finance affirmations and Christian money meditations.

*****

ANTHOLOGY OF CHRISTIAN BIBLE SERMONS

Anthology of Christian Bible Sermons is a compilation of more than 20 Biblical rhema teachings which include:

* A New Christmas Message

* A New Easter Message

* Are You A Flamboyant Fig Tree Christian?

* Biblical Lessons for Purim from Queen Esther

* Can God Help Me If I Am Surrounded By Enemies?

* How Badly Do You Really Want It?

* Seed Words And The Powerful Tongue

* Spiritual AIDS

* The Three Levels Of Getting Lost

* Why Does God Allow Suffering?

* Your Life Is Your Ministry And Your Storm Is Your Message

* A Perfect God, Imperfect People, and Perfect Plans

* We Are Not Ignorant of His Devices

* How to Prepare for a Dangerous Journey

* Yes, God Can

* How to Serve the Body of Christ

* Conduits of God

* Go Back? Stand Still? Move Forward? Drown?

*****

CHRISTIAN SPIRITUAL WARFARE

Christian Spiritual Warfare teaches you the awesome Bible verses you can use as spiritual warfare prayers, Christian affirmations and in your Christian meditation sessions as you fight your spiritual battles.

You will learn how to fight for the following with Bible verses:

* Marriage * Children * Health

* Christian Faith * Christian Ministry

* Country

* Finances * Job * Business

* Peace of Mind * Restoration * Self Esteem * Self Love

You will also learn how to fight against the following with Bible verses:

* Addiction * Temptation

* Being Single * Infertility

* Opposition * Oppression

* Worry * Fear

* Feelings of Condemnation * Confusion

* Danger * Death * Despair * Discouragement

* Impatience * Insomnia * Laziness * Loneliness

* Poverty * Pride * Sadness

* Vengeance * Weakness

* A Foul Mouth * Lying

*****

DARK SKIN DERMATOLOGY COLOR ATLAS

Dark Skin Dermatology Color Atlas is filled with clear explanations and color photos of skin, hair, and nail diseases affecting people with skin of color or Fitzpatrick skin types IV, V, and VI.

Topics covered include Acne Vulgaris, Alopecia Areata, Anal Warts, Angioedema, Aphthous Ulcers, Atopic Dermatitis, Blastomycosis, Blister Beetle Dermatitis or Nairobi Fly Dermatitis, Cellulitis, Chronic Ulcers, Confetti Hypopigmentation, Cutaneous T Cell Lymphoma, Cutaneous Tuberculosis, Dermatitis Artefacta, Erythema Nodosum,

Exfoliative Erythroderma, Gianotti Crosti Syndrome, Hand Dermatitis, Hemangioma, Herpes Zoster, Ichthyosis, Ingrown Toenails, Irritant Contact Dermatitis, Kaposi Sarcoma, Keloids, Keratoderma Blenorrhagica, Klippel Trenaunay Weber Syndrome, Leishmaniasis, Leprosy, Leukonychia, Lichen Nitidus, Lichen Planus,

Lichenoid Drug Eruption, Linear Epidermal Nevus, Linear IgA Dermatosis (LAD), Lipodermatosclerosis, Lymphangioma Circumscriptum, Miliaria, Molluscum Contagiosum, Neurofibromatosis, Nickel Dermatitis, Onychomadesis, Onychomycosis, Palmoplantar Eccrine Hidradenitis, Papular Pruritic Eruption (PPE), Paronychia, Pellagra, Pemphigus Foliaceous,

Pemphigus Vulgaris, Piebaldism, Pityriasis Rosea, Pityriasis Rubra Pilaris, Plantar Hyperkeratosis, Plantar Warts, Poikiloderma, Postinflammatory Hyperpigmentation and Hypopigmentation, Post Topical Steroids Hypopigmentation, Psoriasis, Pyogenic Granuloma or Lobular Capillary Hemangioma, Scabies, Seborrheic Dermatitis, Steven Johnson Syndrome (SJS) and Toxic Epidermal Necrolysis (TEN),

Sunburn, Systemic Sclerosis, Tinea Capitis, Tinea Pedis, Tinea Versicolor, Traction Alopecia, Urticaria, Vasculitis, Vitiligo, and Xanthelasma.

*****